I0436716

Copyright

Disclaimer

Table of Contents

Introduction

After working in the medical field for over 20 years, I have come to appreciate the amazing ability of the human body to work within itself to correct imbalances or to heal injuries. It is a truly miraculous site to see a person come to you as a patient - broken, unwell or barely able to respond and see that person improve to the point of walking down the hall or dressed in their own clothes, ready to leave the hospital with their family. This miracle is one reason I became a nurse. There is satisfaction in helping that person with their journey to better health.

On a personal level, heart disease and Hypertension have taken people close to me. My mother had high BP and was on medication for Hypertension, but this was back in the 1970's and the choice of medications were few. I remember she would comment that she did not like the way she felt when she took her medication, so sometimes she didn't take it. In 1975, she died at the age of 38. My father had a heart attack with coronary artery bypass graft at the age of 63. My family history has motivated me to be mindful of my own health and to be pro-active by watching my diet, exercising and going to regular, annual check-ups with my physicians. My family history has also pushed me to encourage others to be pro-active in their heart health.

Have you ever heard the term "baby steps"? This is when you set small goals for yourself that are easily achievable. Then as you progress through those goals, you set higher and higher goals. By using this method, you are less likely to become discouraged and feel like you have failed. While reading this guide, think of small decisions you can make to your everyday schedule to achieve a healthier lifestyle.

Positive energy and positive attitude go a long way when trying to make healthy changes in your lifestyle. Having family members or friends to encourage you can make a huge impact on the results you can achieve.

"A positive attitude gives you power over your circumstances instead of your circumstances having power over you."

Joyce Meyer

While working in both the ambulatory setting and the hospital setting, Hypertension is one of the most common diagnoses I have encountered. I believe patient education is an important part of preventative medicine………so let's **GET GOING!**

Living with Hypertension

Hypertension (HTN) is called "the silent killer". The reason is simple, most people don't even know that their blood pressure is high unless they happen to get their blood pressure taken at a doctor's office or out in the community at a blood pressure machine or a health fair. Many people don't have any symptoms of elevated blood pressure until after it has started causing damage.

As your blood pressure slowly increases, you go on about your life without any symptoms at all. After years of increasing blood pressure, the toll on your body finally gives you a sign. You may have a headache or a nosebleed, you may feel anxious or short of breath. "It's no big deal, I don't need to go to the doctor for that," you say to yourself.

One day you have a severe headache with shortness of breath. You make an appointment with your doctor and your blood pressure is 188/103 – You're in Hypertensive Crisis. This is a life threatening condition that can lead to a heart attack or stroke.

According to the America Heart Association, there are about 80 million people diagnosed with high blood pressure, also known as Hypertension in the United States. If left untreated, this can have a devastating impact on your body and health. It can also have a financial impact on the healthcare system as well as your wallet. This guide will assist you in gaining control over your HTN and help you to live a healthier, active life.

What Is Hypertension?

The human body has a remarkable network of systems to help keep it in balance. The heart and lungs pump vital nutrients and oxygen laden blood to the major organs such as the brain, liver and kidneys, through the arteries. Veins then return blood that has been depleted of nutrients and oxygen to the heart and lungs to start the cycle over again. In a healthy person, this continuous rotation is done unnoticed in everyday life. As we age, our body systems can become less efficient and/or chronic medical conditions can arise. Hypertension (HTN), or high blood pressure (BP), is a common occurrence due to the aging body. Arteries can become hardened or constricted. Plaque buildup, which can occur due to high cholesterol levels or coronary artery disease (CAD), can make blood vessels diameter smaller. The blood volume in your body then has to circulate through narrowed vessels and causes more pressure to be exerted on the vessel walls. This pressure, when increased, is called Hypertension. Blood pressure is measured in units called mmHg, this stands for millimeter of mercury. There are two numbers that are measured, such as

120/80 mmHg. The top number, the systolic reading, will always be higher than the bottom number. It is the measurement of force placed on the artery wall when the heart pumps. The bottom number, the diastolic reading is the measure of pressure with the heart is at rest.

The increase in force on the vessels, make the heart work harder to pump blood throughout your body. If your blood pressure readings become consistently elevated (greater than 140/90), damage can occur to other body systems that require nutrients and oxygen to maintain homeostasis (balance). Blood pressure is rated in four stages:

Normal

Systolic pressure: below 120 mmHg

Diastolic pressure: below 80 mmHg

Pre-hypertensive

Systolic pressure: 120 – 139 mmHg

Diastolic pressure: 80 – 89 mmHg

HTN – Stage 1

Systolic pressure: 140 – 159 mmHg

Diastolic pressure: 90 – 99 mmHg

HTN – Stage 2

Systolic pressure: 160 mmHg or higher

Diastolic pressure: 100 mmHg or higher

Blood pressure will naturally rise with increased activity, excitement or nervousness. On the flip side, blood pressure will be naturally lower when at rest or during sleep. Having an elevated blood pressure reading one or two times does not mean you have HTN. For a diagnosis of HTN, blood pressure readings will be consistently high over a series of several readings.

Causes of HTN

Hypertension is broken into two types. Primary HTN is defined as having chronic elevated blood pressure readings with no other disease state present. Primary HTN is less commonly diagnosed, but can still cause damage to other body systems if left untreated. Secondary HTN is the most common type of HTN diagnosed and is caused by other chronic diseases such as heart, kidney or lung disease. There are other known factors that can increase the risk of HTN.

Gender can affect blood pressure. Men are more likely to develop HTN before the age of 45. Women are more likely to develop HTN after the age of 65.

Race can also be a risk factor for developing HTN. African-Americans, unfortunately, have a higher chance of developing HTN and it can develop at an earlier age. It is also much harder to control, usually requiring a combination of medications.

Family history of HTN will raise the odds of developing HTN. Your risk of developing HTN is doubled if you have a least one parent with HTN.

Age is another factor, as our age increases, so does the risk of developing HTN.

Some medications can contribute to elevated BP. Here are some commonly prescribed and over-the-counter medications that can increase your BP.

- Oral contraceptives

- Nonsteroidal Anti-Inflammatory agents (NSAIDS)

- Decongestants (cough medications)

- Weight loss medications

- Stimulants

Over the Counter (OTC) medications or herbal supplements can cause blood pressure to rise. Ask your doctor or pharmacist before taking a new OTC or supplement. Some herbal supplements can interfere with HTN medications. Check with your pharmacist for any harmful interactions.

Illicit drugs, or street drugs such as methamphetamines and cocaine make your BP increase as well as cause irreversible damage to the heart.

Effects of HTN

Having a chronically elevated blood pressure can affect other areas of your body. The pressure on the vessels start to damage them and when the blood can no longer flow freely through the vessels, nutrients and oxygen cannot reach vital organs such as brain, eyes, heart and kidneys. HTN is the most common risk factor for both heart attack and stroke.

When blood pressure remains in an elevated state and damages the blood vessels, the walls of the vessels become thick or hard. Plaques can form inside the arteries due to fatty deposits and further narrow the blood flow. When the plaque flakes off it can travel to the heart or the brain and lodge into smaller arteries in the heart or brain. This stops blood flow to that area and can cause loss of oxygen (ischemia) to the heart or brain. The resulting damage to the muscle in the heart is called a heart attack (Myocardial Infarction). If the damage is in the brain, it is called a stroke. Both are considered medical emergencies and immediate medical attention is needed.

HTN long term effects can lead to Congestive Heart Failure (CHF) and Cardiovascular disease. CHF is when the heart is damaged and can no longer function efficiently. Since the heart is not working properly, other organs suffer due to lack of oxygen and nutrients. Cardiovascular disease is when the blood vessels that supply blood to the heart muscle are damaged and reduce blood flow to the pump.

Chronic HTN can also cause weakness in blood vessel walls. Think of your arteries as a bicycle tire, when you put pressure on the tire by over-inflation, it can cause a bulge on the side of the tire. The same can happen to arteries; this is known as an aneurysm. Because this is a weakness in the vessel, there is a chance the aneurysm could rupture and internal bleeding can occur. This is a medical emergency and immediate medical attention is needed.

Your eyes are fed nutrients and oxygen through tiny vessels behind the eye. Because the vessels are so small, it is easy to understand why any constriction can result in decrease of nutrients and damage to the retina which can lead to blindness.

Kidney damage or failure is also common when HTN is not controlled or has been present for a long period of time. Kidneys demand a high flow of blood volume to aid in filtering out toxins in the body through urine. HTN decreases blood flow to the kidneys and damages their filtering abilities, making them vulnerable to failure.

Medications for HTN

Thanks to many years of research and development, there is a large selection of medications that can help to control you BP. These medications are broken down into classes based on how they work. The most widely used classes are angiotensin-converting enzyme (ACE) inhibitors, angiotensin II receptor blockers (ARBs), beta-adrenergic blockers, calcium channel blockers, centrally acting adrenergics, diuretics and vasodilators.

Angiotensin-converting enzyme (ACE) inhibitors – This class contain medications such as captopril, enalapril and lisinopril and are generally called ACE inhibitors for short. Angiotensin I is made in the body and is a weak vasoconstrictor. The term vasoconstrictor means that it constricts the blood vessel, making it more difficult for blood to flow through and increasing blood pressure. Angiotensin I converts to Angiotensin II, which is a vasoconstrictor that causes systemic (entire system) and renal blood vessels to constrict, which again, decreases blood flow and increases blood pressure. ACE inhibitors block the conversion of Angiotensin I to Angiotensin

II so that vessels do not constrict and therefore keeps the BP from rising.

Angiotensin II receptor blockers (ARBs) – This class contains medications such as losartan and valsartan. As stated above, Angiotensin II is a potent and systemic vasoconstrictor. ARBs work by binding Angiotensin II receptor sites in the cells so that Angiotensin II cannot reach the receptor sites and cause constriction. It is kind of like playing musical chairs, if all of the chairs are full, little Angiotensin II has no place to sit and is out of the game.

Beta-adrenergic blockers – This class contains medications such as atenolol, metoprolol, labetolol, nadolol and propranolol and are generally call Beta Blockers. They work by blocking the effects of hormones such as epinephrine or adrenalin, which can make the heart beat stronger and faster. The Beta Blockers block this action so that the heart beats slower and with less force. The result is lower BP and increase blood flow.

Calcium channel blockers – This class contains medications such as amlodipine, diltiazem, nifedipine and verapamil. They work by blocking calcium ion from crossing the cell membrane in the cardiac and vascular smooth muscle. This action allows the muscles to relax and opens up (dilates) the cardiac and vascular vessels so that flow is increased and pressure is decreased.

Centrally acting adrenergics – The most commonly used medication in this class is clonidine. Centrally acting adrenergics work by reducing impulses to the sympathetic nervous system (SNS). The SNS is part of the central nervous system that is in control of the "fight or flight" response. When the SNS system is triggered, blood vessels constrict so that your body is prepared to defend or flee. The medication works to decrease the impulses in the SNS, thus decreasing BP.

Diuretics – This class contains medications such as furosemide, hydrocholorothiazide (HCTZ) and bumetanine and is sometime referred to as a "water pill". There are several sub-groups in this class. These medications are grouped by how they work, but they all have a common goal – to reduce unneeded water and sodium through urination. By reducing excess fluid in the blood volume, pressure inside the blood vessels will be decreased.

Vasodilators – This class contains medications such as hydralazine and minoxidil. They work by relaxing smooth muscles in the arteries, thus open the blood vessels and reducing BP.

The most common side-effect from taking medications for HTN is low blood pressure. If the medication works too well, or too fast you can become dizzy or faint (syncope). When starting new HTN medications be sure to rise from a sitting position to a standing positon slowly to allow your body to adjust while getting use to the new medication. Less common side-effects include slow heartbeat (bradycardia), fast heartbeat (tachycardia), headache or nausea. Some of these effects may only last for a few days. Also read any information given to you about a new medication. If you have any concerns or questions about how to take a medication or what the side-effects can be, talk to your doctor or pharmacist.

Regardless of what prescriptions your doctor recommends, the most important thing to remember is that medications only work when they are taken. Follow the instructions given by your doctor and don't stop or skip any medication without first consulting with him or her. Make sure to refill your medications early so that you eliminate the possibility of running out, especially when planning for a trip or vacation. Medications can help tremendously with gaining control over your HTN, but they can't do it alone. Lifestyle changes, even small ones, can increase your chances of decreasing your BP and controlling your HTN.

10 Simple Steps to Take Control of Your HTN

1. Check Your Blood Pressure

Knowing how and when to check your BP will
help you gain control of you HTN. There are
several BP monitors on the market and they have
several different price points. Some are made for
the arm and others are made for the wrist. Make
sure you find one that is the right size for you and
that is reliable. Measure your arm or wrist with a
measuring tape to ensure a proper fit. Read the
instructions to make sure you are comfortable
with the machine. Try to use the same
cuff/machine each time to get a more reliable
reading. If you switch between public machines
and different home machines, your readings
could be slightly off depending on the machine
used.

Before taking your BP reading, make sure you
remove tight fitting clothes from the area you are
using to take your BP. Relax in a quiet room for
about 10 minutes before attempting to get a BP
reading. When you are ready to take your BP, sit
with your feet on the floor and legs uncrossed.
Having your legs crossed can alter your BP

reading. If possible, have the arm that you are obtaining the reading from stretched out, but relaxed, at the same level as your heart (example: a table). Do not hold your arm up in the air or tighten your arm muscles, this will unnecessarily raise your BP reading.

Place the cuff on your arm, as directed by the manufacturer's instructions. Make sure the cuff is in the correct position and not in the bend of your elbow or wrist. If the cuff has a marking on it such as "artery", make sure it lines up with the artery that runs up the inside surface of your arm, opposite of your elbow. The cuff should be snug but not tight, you should be able to insert a finger between the cuff and your arm to check for a good fit. While the cuff is inflating and taking a reading, stay still but breathe normally, holding your breath may alter the reading. Once you obtain the reading results, document it so that you may see trends in BP readings.

It is usually best to take your BP at around the same time of day, each day. There are exceptions such as you feel like your BP is really high or really low. If this occurs don't hesitate to perform a reading. Document this reading as well as what was happening when you felt your BP was up or down. Your doctor will need to see these results.

2. Control Other Medical Conditions

If you have other medical conditions such as Diabetes, Kidney Disease, or Heart Disease, it is best to keep them under good control. Other chronic medical conditions such as pain, obesity and high cholesterol, can elevate your BP as well. By working with your doctor(s) to control these medical conditions, you will also be taking a step towards controlling your HTN.

3. Diet

The "Dietary Approaches to Stop Hypertension" known as the DASH diet, is a great way to help control HTN. It consists of a diet high in fruits and vegetables as well as whole grains. DASH focuses on eating more fresh fruits and vegetables. If that is too constricting or costly, using frozen fruits and vegetables that have no added salt or sugar can be an alternative. Stay away from processed food such as canned, bagged, jarred or boxed foods. These foods usually use a lot of salts, fats and sugars as preservatives. Frozen ready-made meals, lunch meats or cured meats contain a high amount of salt (sodium).

The DASH diet recommends avoiding salt, red meats and sugar. The recommended salt intake should be lower than 1,500 mg per day. By cooking with herbs, you can decrease the amount of salt intake without losing flavor. Be aware that some spices such as garlic salt, soy sauce and steak sauce contain a lot of salt. Also, foods that advertise "low fat" usually contain a large amount of salt. When they remove fat from the product, flavor suffers so they add salt to make the food more palatable.

When choosing meats, stick to skinless chicken, turkey, fat trimmed pork, fish and seafood. Stay away from red meats that are fat marbled, if you choose to eat red meat make sure it is 85% lean or leaner. Decrease the portion size, instead of eating a 10 ounces, eat 6 ounces, which is about the size of a deck of cards.

If you go out to eat, start with small changes,

then add more as you go along. Reduce the size of your portions or instead of ordering fries and a burger, only order the burger, even better order a grilled chicken sandwich. If you make drastic changes from the start, you are less likely to stick with the lifestyle change over the long haul.

4. Exercise

Exercise can help to relieve stress as well as decrease weight. It has also been shown to improve symptoms of depression. **IMPORTANT:** Always consult with your doctor before starting an exercise program. Doing cardio/aerobic exercise at least 30 minutes, 3-4 days of the week is a great goal to work towards, but don't feel that it is unattainable. Start with baby steps and increase your exercise as your tolerance to the exercise increases. The point is to do more than you are doing now. If you can't run, try to do a fast walk. If you are unable to do a fast walk, start with a slow walk or walking in place while making sure your knees come up as high as you can tolerate. The socialization aspect of exercise can be a benefit as well. Join a gym or join a walking or running club in your area. If there is no club in your area, start one, they are a great source for motivation.

5. Lose Weight

To lose weight, there is one tried and true way to succeed, decrease the amount of calories you take in and increase the amount of calories you burn. There are many types of weight loss plans that can be used. Some options are making an appointment with a nutritionist, join a franchise weight loss program, or if your frugal, like me, search the web for ideas that are tailored to your own needs. When it comes to weight loss the most effective plan is the plan you stick with. This is not a New Year's resolution; this should be a lifestyle adjustment.

6. STOP Smoking

Smoking cigarettes that contain nicotine causes blood vessels to constrict temporarily, which can cause blood pressure to rise. Long term smoking can lead to HTN. According to the American Heart Association, studies have shown the chemicals in cigarettes have been found to cause Coronary Heart Disease (CAD) which narrows the vessels diameter with fatty plaque buildup. A person diagnosed with CAD, who continues to smoke, increases their risk for a heart attack exponentially. To improve your chance of living a longer and healthier life there is only one option – **STOP SMOKING!** There are several online sites or app programs to help you stop smoking. Most states have their own hotline with tips and incentives to stop smoking. Take it one day at a time and if you don't succeed, don't get discouraged, try it again. Take the first step now and let your heart and lungs reap the benefits.

7.   Moderate Alcohol Intake

Heavy consumption of alcohol increases BP and chronic alcohol use can cause HTN. Because alcoholic drinks are usually loaded with calories, it can also lead to unwanted weight gain. If consumed in moderation, alcohol, particularly red wine, has been shown to have positive effects on the heart. Red wine has antioxidants and resveratrol that are found in the skin of the red grapes that make the wine. Antioxidants can help to increase high-density lipoprotein cholesterol (HDL). HDL is the healthy cholesterol in your body that is needed to protect and maintain healthy arteries. Resveratrol has been studied and might help decrease low-density lipoprotein cholesterol (LDL), which is the bad cholesterol that can cause damage to arteries.

Moderation is defined as no more than two drinks a day for men and no more than one drink a day for women.

A drink consists of:

- 12 ounces of beer

- 5 ounces of wine

- 1.5 ounces of 80-proof distilled alcohol

Alcohol can also interfere with some HTN medications.

8. Reduce Stress

Stress has been shown to increase BP. Finding ways to decrease stress is important to help lower your BP. There are several activities that can help lower stress levels. Finding the one that works for you is the best way to ensure lifelong benefits. Some people use meditation or Yoga while others find the social aspect that comes while working out in a gym helps them to relief stress. Studies have proven that having a pet can reduce stress, by petting or "chilling" with your pet, anxiety levels and stress are lowered. Hobbies are another way to control the stress in your life. Carve out a small slice of time in your life to do things that you enjoy and reap the health rewards.

The socialization of group exercise such as a club or gym can help to reduce stress. Spending time with a great friend or a beloved family member has also been shown to reduce stress. It would be best to stay away from negative personalities and drama-filled situations to help reduce stress.

Not getting regular quality sleep has been linked to heart disease, which can lead to HTN. Sleep

10. Collaborate With Your Doctor(s)

A good, trusting relationship with your doctor(s) is important. Since multiple specialties can be involved in your care due to other medical conditions, be sure to have a complete and accurate list of your current medications for each visit. Make sure you keep your appointments and actively participate in your care. Make a list of questions or topics that you want to ask your doctor about during the appointment, so that you don't forget. By keeping other medical conditions under control and working closely with your doctor, you can avoid issues that can derail your chances of taking control of your HTN.

By making some of these lifestyle changes, you can decrease your BP and it may be possible to reduce your HTN medications, or stop them completely. Whatever you tackle first, choose realistic goals and set a deadline.   When you write your goal down, make sure your goal is specific such as: walk 10 minutes a day, instead of writing down exercise more. This will help to keep you on track. Get a partner, such as a family member or friend, who will keep you accountable towards your goal. Make it fun and something to look forward to, instead of a chore, so it will increase your odds of succeeding.

When to Seek Help

It is important to know when you should seek medical attention. Here are some tips on what to look for:

Call your doctor if you have:

- A recurrent headache.

- Dizziness.

- Swelling in your lower legs or feet.

- Problems with your vision.

Seek immediate help if you experience:

- Sudden or severe blurry vision or double vision.

- Sudden or severe headache or confusion.

- Sudden or severe chest pain and/or nausea/vomiting.

- Difficulty breathing.

- Unusual weakness or feel faint.

- Numbness, especially on one side of the body or slurred speech.

- Severe nosebleeds.

Glossary

Aneurysm – an abnormal dilation of a blood vessel, most common in an artery. Can be caused by a defect that is present at birth or a weakness of the wall.

Arteries – blood vessels that distribute oxygen-rich blood to the body and organs.

Atherosclerosis – hardening of the arteries due to deposits of cholesterol, lipids or calcium on the artery walls.

Cardiologist – a physician that specializes in the study of the heart.

Cardiovascular Disease – (CVS) any disease of the heart and/or blood vessels.

Cerebrovascular Accident – (CVA) also known as a stroke is when there is damage to the tissue of the brain due to lack of oxygen because of a vessel blockage.

Congested Heart Failure – (CHF) also called heart failure is when the heart is damaged and can no longer function efficiently. Fluid begins to back up causing congestion in tissues and lungs.

Homeostasis – the act of balancing the internal environment of the body by a constant process of feedback and regulation of electrolytes in response to changes both in and out of the body.

Myocardial Infarction – (MI) also known as a heart attack is when there is damage or loss of living heart muscle due to a lack of oxygen because of a coronary artery blockage.

Primary Care Physician (PCP) – a physician that specializes in general practice such as Family Practice or Internal Medicine.

Sodium – an electrolyte in the body that helps to maintain a healthy balance. Also can be known as common table salt.

About The Author

C. H. Truelove – Registered Nurse with a Bachelor of Science in Nursing – understands the importance and benefits of having the right tools to help achieve a healthy lifestyle. Her passion in the healthcare field, and in particular cardiology, has led her to reach out to others, through written word and blogging, to help people gain the tools they need to improve their overall health and well-being.

With more than 24 years working in the healthcare field and 9 years specializing in heart related conditions, she was motivated to pursue one of her goals to put her specialized knowledge of cardiac medicine to print. By becoming an author, online publisher and blogger, she can reach a wider audience and assist more individuals in their quest for a healthier heart.

She is owned by her dogs: Lucy and Milo – brother and sister Miniature Pinschers, who keep her entertained and moving. She also enjoys playing Pickleball, a new obsession that is a great form of exercise and socialization. Other hobbies include crafts such as crocheting, knitting and acrylic painting. She is an avid couponer and deal finder

and relishes Skyping with family members,
particularly her grandchildren.

Thank You!

Thank you so much for downloading this book!

My hope is that this book will give you accurate information on Hypertension and steps to take to improve your life and HTN. As you take the steps suggested in this book, you will see a noticeable difference.

By taking control of your Hypertension, you will be able to live a more active and healthier life.

Lastly, if you have enjoyed this book, please leave a review on Amazon on the product page where you purchased this book. This kind act will help me to reach more people.

Thank you and good luck with your journey to better health.

But wait! There's more!

You can visit my Website

www.SoundHeartToday.com

There are articles, exercises and heart healthy recipes that will enhance your chances of succeeding in your quest to better health while living with HTN.